HEALTHY N FABULOUS

Eat'n Green N Clean

by MELISSA WILLIAMS

HEALTHY N FABULOUS

EAT'N GREEN N CLEAN

Published by Melissa Williams

Dallas, TX 75235

For more information visit https://www.facebook.com/melissawilliamslosepoundswithme/

DISCLAIMER: AUTHOR does not guarantee that any products or recommendations provided in this book will give you the same benefits or results that she has accomplished. You should consult with a medical doctor or a certified nutritionist before starting any diet program. Please be advised to do your own research to determine if any of the products, information, or suggestions made in this book by the author would work for you. While the author has made every effort to provide accurate information, neither the publisher nor the author assumes no responsibility or liability for personal injury, loss, or damage that may result from suggestions and information in this publication.

The book is sold with the understanding that neither the author nor publisher, is engaged in rendering any legal, financial, medical, or other professional advice. If medical expertise is required, the services of a licensed professional should be sought, as author is not a medical practitioner. By reading this book, you agree to the above disclaimer.

Melissa Williams

ISBN: 13:978-1522713791

ISBN: 10:1522713794

Printed in the United States of America

Table of Contents

Dedicated to everyone,
who wants to get healthy and fabulous.

INTRODUCTION

Congratulations! I am so proud of you for making the decision to take control of your health. Welcome to a new journey in your life. Your body will love the ride to the healthier and fabulous lifestyle of eat'n green and clean.

ROLLER COASTER DIETS SUCK

Don't you just hate the word DIETING? I do. In fact, I run extremely fast when someone mentions diet pills. First thing that comes to mind, is a list of do's and don'ts. Most diet plans are a program that you follow for a period of time. You lose a bit of weight and then gain back more than you've bargained for. Now, that's not fun at all. After spending so much money on fad diets, pills, and drinks myself, I understand the struggle that other women go through. I called this the yo-yo diet. The diet that scams people out of a lot of money based on their catchy advertisements and you still don't lose weight sometimes, but you always lose your money.

I've heard so many stories from clients that had spent so much money on diet pills that didn't work for them. I did the same thing over the years; especially when I wanted the weight off fast, a quick fix. There are some great health products in the market, but there are also some harmful products to be aware of. When I came across the famous "Iaso Tea by Total Life Changes," I have to admit I was skeptical to try it at first because I'd been burned out by scammers. But, for ten dollars, I just gave it a try for the heck of it. I lost a few pounds in the first 5 days, but needed to try the tea again.

Well, the next time I tried the tea again I lost more weight. Now, I was on cloud nine with excitement. Altogether, I lost a total of 22lbs in 3 weeks. I was sold by the amazing results I got from the detox tea and joined the business. The products worked well for me because it was all natural and not toxic to my body. The energy it gave me was just what I needed to get through a hectic day.

Dieting is hard and so many people quit before even losing an ounce of weight.

Why do People Quit Dieting?

- Too expensive to buy products.
- They keep craving for their favorite food.
- Not seeing rapid results quickly.
- Struggle with emotions and rely on food as a comforter.
- Not enough time with a busy life.

Today, you will no longer go on a diet, but you will learn the importance of healthy eating habits. You will learn how to choose your food wisely and portion size control. I don't want you to ever have to focus on counting calories again. Counting calories is hard to keep up with and there's not enough time in the day to keep track of the amount of food you consume. What I want you to get in the habit of doing is learning how to eat healthy and not eat with your eyes. Our eyes can easily be enticed when we see something that looks delicious. We start wishing to have it and talk our minds into buying it because of the appealing look. Many times, we're not even hungry. To avoid this happening to you avoid the deli area and drink some water.

Most every women I know wants to lose weight or their belly bulge, which seems so challenging to do. But, it can be done by adapting to a healthier lifestyle that will change your life forever. Not, only will you lose the weight, but you will be able to maintain the figure. The number one reason why people gain the weight back after losing the pounds is because they go back to their unhealthy eating lifestyle. Everything they did during their diet went out the window. They're just happy that they've dropped a few dress sizes and survived the whole dieting plan. The plan should be to lose it and not gain it back ever again. Eating healthy is not an overnight process; it's a lifetime change. A change that should continue after any program you completed. If not your wasting your time and money.

Now, I'm not saying that you can't have your favorite foods anymore, but you will not crave them like you use to before. Your body has been trained to eat healthy. Just eat small portion size and you will do just fine. If you mess up don't quit just continue on to your journey to a healthy living. Like, I said before this is not a walk, crawl or an overnight process, but a life transformation. In this book, you will find a lot of helpful tips and information that will help you to not only lose the weight healthy, but to keep it off forever.

I'm cheering you on to the finish line and can't wait to hear your testimony of how healthy and fabulous you are.

CHAPTER ONE

WHY YOU SHOULD DETOX BEFORE LOSING WEIGHT

Detox is the first step to take before beginning any weight loss challenge. It is the process of removing toxic substances from the body. Detoxing rids the body of parasites, worms, and toxins. There are several detox methods that exist. While this has not been scientifically proven, detox removes any toxins or parasites from the human body. Many people have shared miraculous stories how they feel more rejuvenating and energetic while they are detoxing including myself. When you're detoxing remember to watch what you eat and drink and to only have foods and liquids that will help to flush out the toxins from your body. Some people have lost a lot of weight during their detox because they are not eating the bad stuff such as processed food and they stay away from the drive-thru lines. Like many low calorie diet plans, detox works for a short period of time, but does not serve as a healthy, or a permanent long time plan.

With any detox, drinking lots of water is crucial to flush the toxins out of the body. Drink at least 8 glasses a day.

My favorite detox tea that has worked well for me is the *Iaso Tea*. It is a natural tea with nine organic herbs. This detox tea is very popular and the natural feeling and energy that you get is amazing. This tea helps eliminate the bloating in your stomach, remove intestinal sludge and parasites. But, find a detox that will work best for you. This is not a treatment for alcoholism or any type of substance abuse. If you're trying to detox from alcohol or substance abuse contact a medical professional. Be mindful that detoxing is not a weight loss diet and should not be overuse. Even if you feel great on your fast, don't continue detoxing for more than 10 to 14 days at max. Long-term fasting or starvation can do irreversible damage to your metabolism. Some detoxes may cause lethargy in the first day or two, so give yourself time to relax and avoid exercise activity during this period. Use this time to mediate and rest.

Here are some great detoxes you can try:

- Green Smoothie- This is one of my favorite detox, and I have lost some weight doing this for ten days. I did the JJ. Smith detox which is a mixture of fruits and vegetables and loved it. I had to tweak it a bit, because too much sugar isn't good. Instead of using four fruits, I used two and it worked fine. The greener the smoothie the better. Now, I know some people don't like the bitter taste from the vegetables so I say experiment, but don't overdo it with the fruits. Many have ask does detox work and my answer is always yes. You just have to be discipline and follow through the process. Do not detox for more than ten days because it can be harmful to the body after a while. As, you detox your body is only getting a small amount of calories so therefore detoxing for a long period of times is not recommended, but consult your doctor first. After, cleansing continue adding vegetables and fruits to your diet. Then, after a week of cleanse gradually start eating again, but eat cleaner and greener so you can be healthier.

- Grapefruit- Is another great detox that many people have tried and love. It is full of natural juices and fiber. The vitamins in this round light colored fruit will help your body to repair from the damage of poor eating. That's why it is known as one of the best nutritional food to eat while cleansing. This fiber-filled fruit will keep you full and rid your body of disgusted waste. Grapefruit has a unique flavor that is bitter yet sweet. While, I don't like the bitter taste of grapefruit, I've learned to suck it up and eat it. It's good for the body. Some people adore grapefruit right off the bat, while others consider it to be an awful nasty taste. The soluble fiber and pectin found in grapefruit helps the digestive system to do its job. Grapefruit juice also helps the body with physical discomfort by

9

relieving heartburn and helping to reduce gas and bloating. You will feel lighter and healthier after dropping a few pounds. You can eat 4-8 grapefruit a day without adding any sugar or sweetener. But, you can add stevia only if you need a little sprinkle of sweet.

- Fruit Detox- Many people do this as a fast without starving themselves. They eat only fruits for a several days. You can eat a variety of fruits, or just have one of your favorite fruit at least six times a day. Having enough fruit will increase your energy because of the natural vitamins and minerals in them. Try apple, grapefruit, orange, blueberries, or grapes. They have an excess amount of Potassium and Vitamin C that does the body good. But, again, you will do well if you eat your favorite foods. After, all who wants to eat fruits that they dislike. Make sure to drink at least eight glasses of water, which I'm sure you already know.

- Liquid Detox- While this is hard to do some people survive this liquid detox. This detox is a liquid only. All you drink is fluids for three days. I wouldn't recommend going any longer than three days. You can drink water with lemon, detox tea any kind you like, or juice fruits and vegetables. Drink lots of liquid to keep your body hydrated. But, make sure when you are juicing that you use lots of greens and fruits so that your body gets all the nourishment that it needs. Some of the vegetables and fruits you can use are:

  ➢ Kale, kiwi, oranges, berries, mango, turnips, spinach, pineapples, apples, grapes, collard greens, celery, peaches, watermelon, grapefruit, banana, carrots, broccoli, parsley and many more to choose from.

CHAPTER TWO

HOW to EAT GREEN and CLEAN?

The increase in obesity is at a massive rate and it's the result of overeating unhealthy food with no nutritional value. Instead of eating low calorie, low fat and natural foods, many of us are, gobbling foods that are loaded with fat, sugar, calories and chemicals. These foods are slowly killing us and does our body more harm than good. The unhealthy foods are causing us to gain weight at rapid speed. What's the answer to this problem? Eat'n green n clean is the answer. More natural whole foods and a nutrient rich diet.

Fruits and vegetables protect our body from chronic diseases. They contain essential vitamins, minerals, and fiber that helps protect you from illnesses, which can be painful, debilitating, and even fatal in some cases. Fruits and vegetables can help to protect against heart disease, stroke, and certain types of cancer, high blood pressure, eye disease and more.

Eating the essential amount of fruits and vegetables can boost your immune system. Your immune system is like a battery. When it's strong, it keeps your car going. And when it's weak, it's dead. A clogged up immune system increases the chances of virus and bacterial, issues such as skin complications, upper respiratory infections, aging and chronic illness. Eating more fruits and vegetables daily is an important key to help boost immune health. You want your immune system to operate regularly and properly. Vegetables and fruits are consumed with fiber, which helps to keep you full longer. Eating fruits and vegetables on your plate, or steamed vegetables and a fruit instead of a dessert gives us the nutrients we need. Fruits and vegetables are not as bad as people make it to be. If you learn to try different ones and not judge them based on looks, you might actually enjoy them.

Unhealthy calories from carbs increase our appetite and weight. Many of us, who love the carbs and are sweet tooth, often struggle with cravings, and emotional eating. This behavior is harmful to our mental and physical health. Eating fruits and vegetables as part of a healthy diet can be an alternative treatment against symptoms, illness, conditions, and even disease. The benefits of eating fruits and vegetables can save us tons of money and time. Less hospital visits and medications. The more fruits and vegetables that we eat on a daily basis the more energize we are naturally without taking energy drinks.

Eating more fresh organic vegetables is one of the healthiest choices you can make to improve your health. Vegetables also help to reduce bloating, and give your skin a more youthful glow

Vegetables are filled with Vitamins, that helps to reduce stress. Eating more green leafy vegetables like spinach, kale, collard greens, parsley are good for people who suffer with stress. These vegetables are packed with magnesium, which balances the cortisol your stress hormones. The vitamin K in vegetables reduces the inflammation in our body. If you suffer from heartburn, eat more vegetables. Magnesium and potassium found in vegetables relaxes the blood vessels, which helps to decrease your blood pressure level. Once you get into a routine of eating healthy, it becomes a habit to you. Like second nature, and you will look forward to your fruits and vegetables. You will look and feel better and healthier. Now start eating your greens so you can live a healthy and fabulous life.

CHAPTER THREE

WHY IS EXERCISE IMPORTANT FOR YOUR LIFE?

Exercise is one of the things many people struggle with the most. Even myself, have a tough time with exercising. I don't like the soreness or pain. In, fact I don't like going to the gym either. But, I've learned that any form of exercise can help keep my body healthy. Not many people can afford a personal trainer or the gym. The number one excuse that people give for not exercising is not enough time in the day or I'm too tired. I am here to share with you that you don't necessarily have to go to the gym to get in shape. But, you have to do some form of exercise.

Exercise helps jumpstart your metabolism. It burns calories. The more you exercise the more calories you burn. Some people burn more calories than others because of their energy level. Your muscles need a lot of energy to burn calories. When you exercise, you sweat and burn calories and fat also.

Exercise is very important, as you get older because you lose muscle mass as you age. Your

16

metabolism slows down. You need to exercise to avoid losing muscle mass. As you age, it's important to protect your bones, joints, and muscles. Not only does exercising support your body and help you to move, but also it keeps your bones, joints, and muscles healthy.

There are tons of exercises that you can do. It's simple. Here is a few exercise that you can try.

- Aerobics is a great workout and gets you sweating those calories off. If you like dancing Zumba is a perfect fit for you. The more intense your work out is the more calories you burn. Get on an elliptical machine and burn that fat off. The gym has a variety of cardio machines to choose from. I say try them all. Remember your muscles will be sore for a few days and that's normal. Everyday challenge yourself to do more. Up your cardio speed and burn more calories. But, don't over work yourself. Move at your own pace.

- Walking around the track, a few times a week, can burn calories. Grab a friend or your kids and go for a walk.

- Running speeds up your metabolism and helps to burn more calories.

- Riding is another exercise you can do. It's cheaper than going to the gym. Ride your bicycle around your neighborhood. The kids will love seeing you go biking with them.

- Run up and down the stairs a few times a day. Yes, this can help you.

- Move around the house instead of calling the kids to get you a glass of water. The more you move around you get your metabolism going.

- Play more with the kids. Children have a lot of energy and running around with them you will burn calories.

- Skip the elevators at work and use the stairs. Taking short cuts will not help you to lose weight. Believe it or not going up those stairs helps strengthens your bones and muscles.

- Do some sit ups, pushups, crunches and squats. Now, I love doing squats it shapes your butt and leg muscles. Crunches are good for your tummy area.

- Start doing stretches daily.

- Get a ball and yoga mat and get to work. You can use your ball to squat with.

- Lift weights. You want to lift some weights to tone your muscles. This helps you to not have loose skin.

- Jump rope. This is a fun exercise for many people to do. Jump ropes are affordable. My brother does this all the time. I am jealous because I can't jump rope at all.

- Jumping jacks is my favorite exercise to do. Do 40 jumping jacks three times a day. If you can do more go for it.

- Find an outdoor sport or activity like volleyball, tennis, hiking, climbing, basketball, or baseball anything you love to do and get your workout going. You will enjoy it more.

- Swimming is a fun exercise. Find a pool or a beach and go for a swim.

Exercising a few times a week will do your body good. Start slow and then gradually increase your workout. But, remember to rest and not over work your body. Your muscles need to repair themselves. So, exercising at a gym four times a week is good enough. You can do some of the simple exercises at home mentioned above.

Physical activity can improve your health and everyone can benefit from it. If you have any medical conditions talk with your doctor before starting any physical activity.

BENEFITS of EXERCISE

- Reduces the risk of heart disease and stroke that are one of the leading causes of death in America. Any type of physical activity can lower your blood pressure and improve cholesterol.

- Regular physical activity can decrease your risk of developing type 2 diabetes. If you have type 2 diabetes doing a moderate exercise will help to control your blood glucose.

- People who are more physical active have a lower risk of developing colon cancer than people who are not active.

- Research has shown that women who are physically active have a lower risk of developing breast cancer, than do people who are not active at all.

- Exercising reduces stress. It is a stress relief. After a long stressful day go for a walk and you will feel a lot better. Go for a run or head to the gym. You will forget that you were even stressed after a good workout. So, when you find yourself about to get into an intense argument go for a walk and it will calm you down and you can think better. I love hitting a punching bag when I'm stress or mad and it works perfect for me. Getting a good workout can help manage physical and mental stress.

Exercise also increases your concentration. Your brain functions better when you're not stressed. Now, you can get sweaty and reduce your stress at the same time.

- If you have anxiety or depression, exercise will help you. Running a few miles on a treadmill can keep your depression under control. Exercise releases endorphins, which create feelings of happiness and euphoria. Try some exercising before taking antidepressant medications. Exercising can boost your mood and help make you feel more joyful.

- Improves your appearance. It boosts your self-esteem. It keeps your body in shape, shred pounds, and looking fine. You not only look good, but you feel fabulous also.

- If you have arthritis, exercising a few hours a week can help to improve your daily tasks and control your pain. As people get up in age, their muscle mass starts to decrease and, their activity levels also. It's important to increase and maintain muscle mass through exercise training, because it helps with strength and balance. You have a better life when your pain free.

- Longevity you live longer when your body is in good health.

- Exercise keeps your weight under control. When you are physically active, you don't gain a vast of amount of weight. Instead, you maintain your weight, figure, and sexy body.

- Exercise spices up your sex life. The more energize you are the better you will be in the bedroom. A person that is physically active is less likely to suffer from sexual dysfunctions. Your body will love a good workout and so will your spouse.

CHAPTER FOUR

HOW TO LOSE WEIGHT and KEEP IT OFF?

Losing weight is not a microwave quick fix, so it takes time. But, it can be done with commitment, dedication, and change. Now, are you ready to get healthy and fabulous? I hope your answer is YES. Let's try this losing weight one more time and keep it off forever. Tell fat good-bye and hello to a new healthier you.

- To lose weight physically the first step is to want to do it mentally. Are you losing weight for you or for others? Losing weight should be for you first. Once you set your heart to do it and why you truly want to get healthy you will try hard and get results.

- Remove all the foods that are unhealthy from the pantry and the refrigerator.

- Discuss with your family what you're trying to do. Get them involve because

24

it makes it a lot easier when the whole house is on the same page. Now, you're thinking it's not fear to my family to eat what I eat. But, you want your whole family to embark this journey to eat healthy and choose a healthier lifestyle. For, example, ask your family to not bring outside food in the house like junk food, sodas, and candies. If it's not in the home, you can't eat it. Like, I always stress everything is in moderation, so it's a good practice to teach your children having junk food every day is not healthy. Explain to them that in the long run it's not good for their health.

- Get the family engaged to help you with the grocery list. Keep the list green n clean as possible. Make smoothies together it is fun and exciting.

- You need to limit your calorie intake to lose weight. Keep in mind that cutting back on calories doesn't mean starving yourself. Many people brag about doing this and it's not good for your body. Yes, you will lose the weight, but you will gain it back double. Not, eating messes with your metabolism, which you need in order for your body to break down the fat. Starving your body can signal to the brain that your body is lacking nutrition and will hold onto to the fat in your body. It can also cause you to lose muscles instead of fat, which is unhealthy. You want to lose fat not muscle. Your body will eventually shut down and you can collapse and get sick. Starving is not the solution, but eating small portions of healthy food is the key. Remember that if you starve yourself you can still gain weight although you are eating less. So, eat at least five times a day. Now, you will not eat five full meals a day, but you will snack in between your meals. Have an apple, celery, grapes, berries, almonds, boil egg, cucumbers, kale, unsalted peanuts, carrots, broccoli, tomatoes, as a snack. There are plenty more healthy snacks to choose from these are just a few.

• Eating breakfast kicks in your metabolism. Most people don't eat breakfast or have the time to. Breakfast is the most important meal of the day because you want to have energy to face your busy day. You may not have time to cook a hot meal in the morning, but find a quick grab and go for breakfast. A fat free yogurt, almonds, fruit, or a smoothie. One cup of oatmeal with almond milk and a teaspoon of honey is great for breakfast. You can fancy it with some fruit or nuts on the top. Now don't overdo it. Make sure that your breakfast is fresh and not package. Try some egg omelet with spinach, peppers and onions use natural seasoning and olive oil a teaspoon.

- Lower the amount of carbs that you eat. This is hard to do because we love our bread, pasta, sauces, and all that good stuff that makes our food taste delicious. These same carbs are what's packing on the pounds. Yes, I hate it too, because two of my favorite foods to eat are macaroni n cheese and pasta. That was hard for me to give up and eat it once in a while. I understand the struggle believe me I do. But, the tough question I had to ask myself was do I want the food that will make me sick or do I want a healthy life.

Well, of course, I choose to be healthy instead, but I do eat it when I have cravings for it. Not, keeping those carbs in the house can help you out a lot. It's that simple. You don't have it; you don't eat it. I had to learn to crave for healthy foods and buy the ones that I enjoy more. Learning to eat healthy was a big struggle for me because many vegetables and fruits that I eat today I've never even heard of them before until now. Although, I'm looked on like the healthy maniac I wouldn't have it any other way, because I want to live a healthy life.

While, you're trying to lose weight stay away from those carbs. They turn into fat and you don't want that. Eat the carbs that are better for you like vegetables. No white rice, pasta, sauces, ketchup, bread mayonnaise, are some examples of what not to eat while losing weight. Carbs are not all that bad, but we tend to have too much which makes it not good for us. For, instance eating three pieces of fried chicken smothered with ketchup for lunch and two pork chops for dinner with potato salad, rice, bread, cake, soda, and chips for snack. That's too much unhealthy carbs. Eat have of your plate with vegetables and without butter. Use only coconut oil, or olive oil, grape seed oil to cook with. Steam your vegetables instead. When you have reached your goal, then you can gradually start adding it back to your daily diet slowly and in moderation. Carbs are tasty just learn to portion size your food.

- Eating enough protein. The body needs protein to maintain lean muscle. Vegetables have a lot of protein such as, kale, broccoli, artichokes, split peas, chick peas, kidney beans, spinach, edamame, black beans, lentils, asparagus to name a few. Eating 4oz of protein with your meals like turkey, fish, shrimp, tuna, eggs, nuts, lean meat, chicken breast, peanut butter unsweetened, low fat yogurt, pumpkin seeds and tofu.

- Sleep is important on your weight loss journey because our bodies need to rest after a long and tiring day. Getting sufficient and adequate sleep is crucial to your physical and mental health. We live longer when we take care of our bodies. When people are restless, they are fatigued, grumpy, moody, and not friendly. Lack of sleep will make you feel sluggish and slow down your metabolism. I am not the nicest person when I'm sleep deprive. You want to get at least 6-8 hours of sleep. Don't neglect your body of rest because you will regret it later on. Your weary and exhausted body will shut down. No one wants to feel like a crump a lump all day. Rest your body and don't fall for the myth "I'll sleep when I die."

- Controlling your stress. It is so easy to get distracted and stressed out when you fail or messed up. Even, if you cheated don't get worked up over it just take a deep breath and start again. Learn how to manage your stress by engaging in fun activities, taking quality time out for yourself. Going for a spa day is also a great treat. Get your hair or nails done. We all need a pampering every now and then. Stay away from negative people.

Surround yourself with people that will make you laugh. If you are stressed and ignore the signs, it can affect your health and cause problems such as physical pain, depression, anxiety, heart disease, and much more complications. Stress can cause you to gain excess weight because you turn to bad habits, such as junk food and you lose control of what you're eating. When people are stress they don't think straight and make poor choices based on their emotions. I encourage you to get the help that you need to live a stress free life. Yoga and daily meditation is a great start. You make healthier eating choices when you're not stressed.

- Exercising and changing your diet. Reducing your calorie intake and combining regular physical activity will help you to not only drop the weight, but to keep it off. After, all who wants to gain the weight right back. Keep in mind that both exercise and a healthy eating plan goes hand in hand. You need both to get the results that you are looking to attain. The more you move the more calories you burn and the quicker your weight drops off. Put on your cardio DVD and get to work.

- It can be a challenge to stay motivated and on track when trying to lose weight. The temptations are always staring you in the face. Let friends know not to bring foods around you that you can't have. Another way to avoid this issue is by staying away from people that will distract you from achieving your goals. Find friends that will support you on your journey and even become your workout buddies. Nothing like a great accountability partner. You will push even harder because you will want to prove a point to your friends that you can accomplish losing weight. Do not allow any to encourage you to skip workouts.

- Get a journal to keep track of what you eat and a record of your exercise. This becomes very helpful and you can see your mistakes and make the necessary changes to do better. You can also use an app to keep track of your calorie intake. A fitness tracker can monitor your steps, calories, and exercise. There are many fitness tracker online to choose from. It is a huge bonus to have because of a busy day it is hard to keep up with what you eat. Now, with this amazing device you can now see where the pounds are coming from.

- Preparing your meals at home saves you a lot of money. Start carrying your lunch and snack to work. Have your lunch prepared the night before.

- Join weight loss groups on social media. These small groups can be very supportive and an encouragement to you while on your weight loss journey.
- Replace your bad eating habits with healthy ones. Make a long-term healthy lifestyle change. Plan your meals in advance this saves you from panicking and buying a quick processed meal. Chew your food slowly so that it can digest properly. When you chew your food slower, you get full faster.

Before You Eat, Ask Yourself These Questions

- Am I really hungry?
- Are vegetables on my plate?
- Am I eating something healthy?
- Am I over eating?

The more you're aware of your actions, the less likely you are to eat out of boredom, emotionally eat, and snack throughout the day. Soothing your emotions with food will leave you feeling worse, which can lead to you putting on weight instead of losing it. Long-term weight loss is much more than a diet. It is a life style change.

However, there are people that can eat whatever they want, and never gain any pounds, while others simply look at food and gain 10 pounds. Now, that's not fair. But, such is life. If you're gaining weight very quickly, it clearly means that your metabolism is slow and you need to boost it up by exercising.

The faster your metabolism, the more calories you burn per day, and the easier it is to lose weight. The slower your metabolism is, the less calories you will burn. And the harder it will be to lose weight. To lose weight you need to speed up your metabolism. There are natural ways to speed up your metabolism without buying those energy drinks just eat healthy foods. Change what you feed your body with bottom line. Healthy foods are the goal to a healthy body and life. Here are some heathy foods that you can add to your diet to help make you feel better and speed up your metabolism.

- Peanut butter, berries, apples, oatmeal, almonds, chicken breast, turkey, vegetables, green tea, water.

The main goal is to nourish your body with healthy foods and exercise and you will lose weight.

CHAPTER FIVE

BENEFITS of Eat'n Green N Clean

- Grape fruit- can help to speed up the process to lose weight. It contains a high amount of fat burning enzymes. Not only does grapefruit increase your metabolism and burn fat, it also gives you all the energy that you need. That's why many people use grapefruit as a cleanse because of its great benefits. It reduces fever. The next time you have a fever eat a grapefruit. Grapefruit helps to provide relief to those suffering from arthritis and joint pain. It lowers your cholesterol and promotes digestion. It boosts your immune system. Feel like you're coming down with a cold have a bite of grapefruit. This is a great fruit to have especially in the winter seasons. The antioxidants found in grapefruit reduce heart disease. This fruit can also help to enhance your outward appearance. Your skin complexion looks more glowing because of the Vitamin C.

- Avocado- Helps the body to produce antioxidant needed for the liver to filter out harmful substance. Avocados are loaded with folate than any other fruit. Folate is important for the brain. Avocado is a food that helps to relieve stress. It is also has natural fats in it. It controls high blood pressure, diabetes and prevents stroke.

- Ginger- Is great for boosting your metabolism and is a natural pain reliever and anti-inflammatory. You can add a ½ teaspoon to a cup of water.

- Garlic- Raw garlic has many health benefits; one is its assistance to liver detoxification. It helps to fight off viruses and bacteria.

- Bragg's Vinegar- Acts like a general toner for your body and especially for the digestive system. It soothes the digestive issues, has antibiotic effects, prevents indigestion, and aids in weight loss. The acetic acid suppresses the appetite. It also reduces the water retention and helps your body burn fats. Apple cider vinegar lowers blood sugar also. You can clean with this vinegar in your home especially if you're allergic to chemical smells. Put a cap full of vinegar into your water first thing in the morning. I love mines warm and Bragg vinegar is natural and not diluted. You can make your salad dressing using this vinegar with some olive oil and natural herbs you like to cook with. Now, you have your own homemade salad dressing without sugar or preservatives.

- Mint Leaf- Is great for aiding in digestion. You can add 10 leaves to your drinking water. It helps to flush toxins from the kidneys, liver, and colon. You can add a fruit for a better taste like blueberries and raspberries or any fruits you wish.

- Peppermint- Alleviates the intestines. It soothes aching toothaches. Increases your memory. I probably can use a bottle a day myself to help me with my memory. Peppermint relieves stress, headaches and rejuvenates you. When you have a headache just put some peppermint oil on your forehead. The next time you are overwhelmed, depressed, stress or just plain moody take a nice hot soaking bath with some peppermint oil. Light some candles and play some meditation or jazz soft music. This will help to make you feel a lot better. Peppermint helps to fight asthma. It even comforts baby colic. If your baby is crying having colic pain, give them a drop of peppermint oil or add it to a little water. Warm water with a teaspoon of peppermint can curb your appetite. A glass of peppermint water can eliminate bloating, give you healthier looking skin, and clean out your kidneys. Peppermint also assists with digestion. You can drink peppermint as a detox also to help flush out the toxins from your body. All you need is a gallon of water, 6 slice of lemon, 1 tablespoon of ginger grated, 10 slices of cucumbers, 12 fresh peppermint leaves. Let your water steep for 8 hours in the refrigerator. Always make a fresh gallon of detox water daily. Never use for more than one day. You can add some blueberries for flavor.

- Natural Honey- This can be use on cuts, burns, mosquito bites, and itchy skin. Honey is excellent for coughs and relieves sore throat. It even fights off infections. Every home should have some honey. For coughs and sore throats, you can drink a cup of warm water, 1 lemon and 2 tablespoon of honey to help relieve the symptoms. Honey helps to boost energy, fatigue and aids in weight loss. You can drink a glass of warm water, a spoon of apple cider vinegar, and a tablespoon of honey with a teaspoon of cinnamon. Honey can be used as a sweetener in your beverages instead of refined sugar. It helps with acne and rubbing your face with it can dry up your acne because it pulls out all the impurities out of your skin.

- Coconut Oil- Helps with weight loss because it doesn't store as fat. It assists in controlling blood sugar, skin eczema, lowers cholesterol, and reduces the risk of heart diseases. It is a stress relief and very soothing for the body. Coconut oil can be used as a moisturizer for the skin and hair. I use it myself. It provides nutrients, nourishment, and protein to your hair allowing it to grow. Massage therapists use this as a massage oil for the body. This oil is good for cooking because it has natural fats. You can deep-fry some delicious fried chicken with coconut oil that will make you slap your momma. I'm just teasing.

- Green Smoothie- Aids in weight loss, healthier looking skin, stabilizes blood sugar levels, reduces risk of diseases, suppresses appetite, natural energy booster, and relieves constipation.

- Green Tea- Helps to fight cancer, strengthens teeth, eliminate bad breathe by reducing bacteria in the mouth, speeds up metabolism, lowers cholesterol, prevents diabetes. Green tea aids in weight loss because it curbs your appetite. This tea also detoxes the body.

- Warm lemon water- Reduces heartburn, body acidity, purifies blood, boosts immune system, lowers blood pressure, improves the liver functions; reduce skin wrinkles and blemishes. It soothes sore throat.

- Cinnamon- It can lower blood sugar levels, reduce heart diseases, help treat muscle spasm and ant-inflammatory. Reduce the risk of colon cancer. It boosts brain function. Great source of calcium to help fight off colds and flu. Cinnamon alleviates gas, indigestion, and nausea. It adds a freshness to stinky breath. Excellent for women who have menstruation cramps. It is a natural pain relief for headaches and arthritis. Cinnamon adds flavor to your beverages and desserts. Many people love baking with cinnamon. Using too much cinnamon on a regular basis can be toxic. Cinnamon can help burn fat. Drink a glass of warm water, honey and a stick or a teaspoon of cinnamon mix together.

- Fruits- Eating fruits in the morning for breakfast can give you a bowel movement before you start your day. The fiber consume in fruits cleanses your colon. Having a lot of fruit can keep your brain energized.

  ➢ Grapes improve your bloodstream levels, which reduces blood clots. It is good for asthma.

  ➢ Cherries contain an antioxidant called cyanide that protects the body from cancer cells.

  ➢ Pineapples help to digest food and build sturdy bones.

  ➢ Apples can lower your cholesterol. It's to fight infections.

  ➢ Watermelons liberate the body of extra ammonia and heal wounds.

  ➢ Banana reduces depression. It gives you natural energy boost. Eating banana can give you healthy bones. It also relieves heartburn and menstrual cramps.

➢ Mangoes help to prevent cancers. It also improves vision, memory, and digestive system.

➢ Blueberries help to protect your heart. It is loaded with antioxidants and cuts belly fat.

➢ Pears boost your immune system.

➢ Cantaloupe is good for the eyes. It reduces fever, high blood pressure and helps with constipation.

➢ Oranges keeps your skin looking young and vibrant because of its natural oil.

➢ Apricots controls blood pressure.

➢ Strawberries heal and strengthen the gums and clean the body out of toxins.

➢ Beets controls blood pressure.

➢ Broccoli helps to strengthen bones and is a great snack you can eat raw. It even lowers cholesterol, and rids the body of toxins.

➢ Cabbage prevents constipation.

- ➤ Chestnuts assist with weight loss. It lowers cholesterol.
- ➤ Carrots are excellent for eyesight.
- ➤ Artichokes aids in digestion.
- ➤ Black beans are good for the heart.
- ➤ Cauliflower protects against prostate cancer.
- Low-fat plain yogurt has probiotic, which helps to relieve digestive complications. It is high in protein and low in fat. Yogurt can help to maintain weight. You can have unsweetened yogurt and add natural honey to sweeten. Make sure watch out for the sugar in yogurts.
- Tuna is high in protein. It is low in calories and fat. Tuna is filled with omega-3 fatty acids that have great antioxidant benefits. You can eat tuna straight out of the can with some lemon. Tuna is delicious on top of a salad.
- Beans help to prevent constipation. It is filled with protein.
- Flaxseed regulates the bowel movement. It is loaded with protein, Omega-3, and fiber. Lowers blood pressure and cholesterol.

Flaxseed also reduces sugar cravings, balance hormones, promotes weight loss because it makes you fuller, improves digestion, and burns fat. It cleanses the colon and nourishes your hair and skin.

- Egg Whites are a great source of Leucine, an amino acid used for weight loss. This amino acid kick starts your metabolism as it raises your base metabolic rate and boosts your weight loss. Be careful when consuming egg whites and avoid eating it raw. There are serious health risks associated to raw egg whites - take the time to cook it and see the health benefits kick in.

- Spinach is high in fiber, which helps to keep you full, protein, iron, Vitamin C &A. It's low in fat and calorie, but high in nutrients. This green leafy vegetable lowers high blood pressure, and strengthens vision. It helps fight diseases, acne, and wrinkles. It also prevents constipation and aids in digestion. This is a great food to help speed up your metabolism and make your skin look healthy and young.

- Chickweed is a vegetable that relieves constipation and helps colon cleansing.
- Mango is an orange looking fruit that helps to relieve constipation.
- Milk is high in calcium, Vitamin D, and protein, which helps to maintain strong bones and teeth. Milk helps with digestion and is a natural antacid. Fat free milk and fat free yogurt can add calcium to your body. Drink more organic, skim, almond milk. Almond milk is a great alternative for people with soy and lactose allergies like myself.
- Aloe Vera detoxes the body. Lowers cholesterol and blood sugar. It supports your immune system. Aloe Vera doesn't have the best taste, but it can also be used for burns, acne, eczema, psoriasis and hydrating the skin. It helps to grow your hair, relieve sinuses, chest congestion, heart reflux, and colds. You can add a few small pieces to some cold water and

let it steep. Honey is a must have to help with yucky taste. Oh, and a mint after drinking.

- Whey is an ideal protein powder for boosting metabolism. It is digested quickly and can help to burn extra calories. Adding some whey into your smoothie can boost your metabolism quickly.

- Oatmeal is a super food for breakfast to jumpstart your metabolism. It is rich in fat-soluble fiber, which requires a lot of energy to break down. This helps boost your metabolism as it also decreases your cholesterol levels and reduces your risk of heart disease.

- Protein helps to build muscle mass.

- Kale is low in calorie, detoxes the body and rich in fiber.

- Cucumbers are high in water and low calorie. It can be eaten as a snack or in salads.

- Parsley cleanses the liver and detoxifies the body.

- Celery is low in calorie, high in fiber and water. It can be eaten as a snack and in salads.

- Almonds decrease food cravings and are rich in fiber.
- Prunes relieve constipation.
- Soybeans have more protein than any other beans. It promotes the digestive system.
- Lentils are loaded with fiber and iron. This vegetable can be cooked in soup or in a salad.
- Peas are an excellent source of protein and can help to reduce the risk of heart disease.

Benefits of Drinking Water

- Relieves headaches. Sometimes headaches are cause by dehydration.
- Flush out bacteria and waste from the body.
- Relieves constipation.
- Healthy looking skin.
- Reduces wrinkles.
- Proper circulation of nutrients in the body.
- Helps to fight of infections and flushes out toxins in the body.
- Prevents urine infections and kidney stones.

- Reduce cold sores, allergies, and colds.

- Keeps your bowels regular.

- Improves your concentration. Not enough water can cause your brain energy level to decline.

- Boosts your energy.

- Keeps you hydrated so that you can function properly. Lack of water can make you feel moody, lazy, and tired.

- Supports the heart.

- Weight loss. Drinking lots of water decreases your appetite.

The benefits of eating fiber are to keep your bowel movements regular, lower cholesterol, and prevent constipation and bowel cancer. Fiber is very important for your health, but also can cause problems if you're already having intestinal complications. Fiber in vegetables and fruits helps to keep you fuller, which aids in weight loss.

Vegetables can help to reduce bloating in your stomach. Not chewing your food properly, eating too fast, overeating can cause bloating. Eating vegetables hydrates your skin, and make you look even more beautiful. It gives you healthy bones. Many people don't like vegetables, but here is a good way to get your vegetables in your body. You can trick your picky eating kids by doing this also. Juice your vegetables and fruit. It is the easy way to get all of your daily vegetables and fruits. You can use a variety of fruits and vegetables. You will get natural energy from your juice.

Eating fruits in the morning for breakfast can give you a bowel movement before you start your day. The fiber consume in fruits cleanses your colon. Having a lot of fruit can keep your brain energized.

Foods high in protein.
- Meat
- Fish
- Eggs
- Dairy products
- Soy
- Nuts

- Chicken
- Shrimp
- Pumpkin seeds, hemp seeds

High protein vegetables.

- Lentils
- Soybeans
- Peas
- Asparagus
- Kale
- Egg plant
- Collard greens
- Broccoli
- Parsley
- Spinach
- Black beans
- Turnips
- Mustard greens
- Watercress

Foods high in fiber. Eating more fiber foods can help to relieve constipation.

- Prunes
- Blueberries
- Peas
- Yogurt probiotic

- Flaxseeds
- Hempseeds
- Chickpeas
- Nuts, Almonds, Pecans
- Squash
- Celery
- Egg plant
- Water

Foods to lower High blood pressure.

- Skim milk
- Spinach
- Green beans
- Banana
- Sunflower seeds
- Soybeans

Foods to avoid that cause high blood pressure.

- Salt
- Processed Foods
- Sodas, artificial drinks
- Sugar

- MSG
- Fast food
- Bacon

Types of Processed Foods

White rice, Bread, Muffins, Grits, Pasta, Pizza, Cake mix, Cookie dough, Pie filling, Jam, Canned foods, Salad dressing, Refined oils, Margarine, Frozen foods, Condiments, Juices, Canned soups, Canned fruits, Lunch meat, Canned meat, Cornmeal, Junk foods such as cookies, chips, Ice cream, Precooked foods, Cheese, Yogurt, Noodles.

CHAPTER SIX

HEALTHY TIPS

- Eating dark green leafy vegetables every day can help to prevent the body from developing cancerous cells and heart disease.
- Fruits and vegetables that are light in color such as tomatoes, carrots, watermelon, cantaloupe, and apricots contain lots of vitamins that help to fight various diseases in the body.
- Add a slice of fruit to your yogurt.
- Make healthy homemade soups with fresh vegetables and freeze it. No can vegetables or tomato soup.
- Always have a side salad of lettuce, cucumber, tomato, pepper, and onion with your meal. You can add one egg.
- Make your own salad dressing. Use apple cider vinegar, olive oil, herbs or red wine, and herbs.
- Eat two different vegetables with your dinner.

- Have a fruit salad or a fruit for dessert instead of a cake.

- Wash your fruits and vegetables with water before eating to remove insects, dirt, and pesticides. You don't want to eat no insects. Do not over wash vegetables because you will be washing away the nutrients.

- Over cooking your vegetables too much, you cook out all the nutrients that your body needs.

- Drink eight glasses of water daily. If you are very active and workout you should drink at least 10 glasses of water. Add some flavor to it if you like, mango, apples, cucumbers, mint or peppermint leaf, ginger and much more.

- Have a fruit and smoothie for breakfast. You can even have a smoothie for lunch. Switch up the ingredients.

- Grapefruit can help you to lose weight. Eat five grapefruits a day as a meal replacement. You can also juice grapefruit and have a few glasses a day. You can juice it with some flaxseed to make you full.

- You can add berries, banana, almond, or pecan to your oatmeal. One tablespoon of fruit. Use only stevia for sweetener. Be careful of the amount of fruit you use.
- Eat less carbs and healthier ones like vegetables and fruits.
- Drinking water naturally reduces your appetite. Having a glass of water before your meals will help you to eat less. A lot of people confuse feeling thirsty with hunger, so they eat when their body is dehydrated. When you're dehydrated, fat cells become harder to break down and so anyone actually trying to diet will find it a lot difficult if they don't drink very much water.
- Add lettuce, sliced tomato, cucumber to your sandwich. Another great way to make sure that you're getting some vegetables in your tummy.
- Eat a couple of dried fruit snacks instead of chips or chocolate.
- Stay away from salt and foods that are high in sodium and alcohol. It can cause you to

develop high blood pressure due to a large amount of sodium intake and low potassium intake from not eating enough fruits and vegetables. High blood pressure complications are mainly because of the foods that we eat. Changing your diet and reducing calories will help to lower your high blood pressure. Foods high in sodium causes high blood pressure, so people should avoid anything with more than 500 mg per serving.

- Use Sea Salt or Mrs. Dash instead of regular salt. Cook with herbs that are more natural for seasoning your food.

- Foods that are processed in a laboratory like margarines are made with hydrogenated oils. Use olive oil, coconut oil, or sesame oil.

- Foods that are high in trans-fat or saturated fats stay away from them. It's simple; avoid fried or fatty foods and the drive thru.

- Foods such as red meat can cause high blood pressure due to toxic substances and chemicals digested by the animals prior to processing.

One of the most ignored facts about high blood pressure is that the complications often occur simply because of the foods you eat. Reducing toxic and calorie intake will lower your high blood pressure.

- Processed foods such as frozen meals, canned soups or any food that's already package should be avoided by all means because they are high in fat and sodium. The estimate sodium intake daily should be between 1500-2500mg. The fat allowance intake should be based on the amount of calories that you eat multiply by 20% then divided by 9 (1200 calories x 20% =240/9=27 grams). This will give an estimate amount of fat you should consume a day. The majority of processed foods are unhealthy. They are very low in nutrients and extremely high on calories. They also contain laboratory chemicals ingredients that can be very harmful to your body. While processed food is a quick convenience eliminating it from your diet can be very challenging. One of the ways to avoid buying a lot of processed food is to purchase a cookbook to help you cook meals. Most people who eat a lot of frozen foods are usually college students, teens and people that are not good at cooking or simple don't like too. Keep in mind that these foods will cause health issues in the future, because it is packed with sugar, fat, and sodium. Which can lead to weight gain, heart problems and blood pressure, putting you at a risk for stroke.

- Stay far away from fast foods restaurants as much as possible. The foods are packed with sodium, trans fat, and carbs. The grease is enough to give you cholesterol.

- If you like alcohol beverages keep in mind that too much can cause high blood pressure. Drink on special occasions if you have to no more than two glasses. If you're detoxing or dieting, you should not drink any alcohol. It has no nutritional value.

- Sodas are not good for your health. Many people love the taste of sodas. Sodas have no nutritional value. All it is a can filled with empty calories and high fructose corn syrup, which is a sweetener that's worse than regular sugar. Sodas are one of the leading causes for obesity. Those dyes in sodas are harmful to our bodies. People who drink more sodas per day have twice the risk of developing heart disease. The caramel color in sodas also causes inflammation. Sodas are high in sodium content, which has been linked with higher risks of a variety of heart problems. The high rate of sodium in soda disrupts the mineral balance by draining potassium and magnesium from the body, which contributes to increased risk for heart diseases. Antacids in sodas can cause constipation, nausea, vomiting, headaches, and kidney damage. Sodas stain your teeth.

- Avoid added sugars. Foods that are loaded with sugar are also high in calories. This causes you to gain weight. Consuming too much sugar on daily basis can put you at a greater risk for heart disease, and diabetes. Make sure that you read the food labels that you purchase for the nutritional information. Watch out for those added sugars in sauces, bread, and salad dressing. Don't buy anything with high fructose corn syrup in it.

- Start a garden in the back yard. I remember my mother always planting a garden in our back yard and it was a lot of work. But, in the end, it saved us money from buying fruits and vegetables at the store and even gas for the car because we didn't had to go anywhere. Just a walk to the back yard garden and picking a ripe tomatoes or pepper. Now, I understand the importance of having a garden. A friend even taught me how to plant vegetables in a pot. Now, that was fun to do except for getting dirt in my fingers. I even learned how to plant Aloe Vera in a pot and use it on my hair to grow it. Some whether seasons permits you from planting a garden now you can do it inside of your house in a plant pot. This is something that you can do with your children.

- Visit your local farm or farmers market and buy some fruits and vegetables. You can get awesome prices.

- The next time you go shopping put your vegetables and fruits on top of the fridge shelf. This makes it noticeable to see it. Put your vegetables and fruits for snack in little containers. I like using the colorful ones for convenience so I can put my veggies in different containers and fruits in another. This makes it a lot easier and saves me time from looking into each container to see which is fruit and vegetable. You can also buy colorful labels to put on your containers.

- Some days frozen fruits and vegetables may be your only options. They are often picked during the winter season and are frozen at the farm. This can be a substitute if you run out of fresh fruits and vegetables.

- Drink half of your bodyweight in ounces of water. If you weigh 120lbs, drink 60oz of water each day. As, you lose weight you can change your water intake.

- Carrying a large bottle of water with you can remind you to drink water. You can be creative with your bottle of water by writing time on it just to remind you to drink up. I called this the water motivation. You can even buy a nice bottle water with motivations on it. There are tons of them online.

- Set an alarm to remind you to drink water. Set alarm every hour or 2 hours because sometimes we can get very busy and forget. Doing this can be a great help to you. You can do this method with your dinner and snacks. Being organized, balanced, having structure and a daily routine is very important and can be a success in your weight loss.

- Make sure to eat raw fruits and vegetables so that you can get all the nutrients from it. Vegetables and fruits are compact with water also so you're not only eating vegetables, but getting some water also. Stay away from those dips or make your own with some grated cucumber or carrots, herbs, cottage cheese, low fat milk. You can use apple cider as dip also yummy.

- Keep healthy snack bars, nuts, and water in your car at all times.
- If you can putting away large plates helps to control how much you put on your plate. Try using salad plates.
- Keep yourself occupied and busy this helps to not focus on food.
- Limit your TV time as much as possible to avoid snacking. When we watch television, we tend to eat all the bad foods like popcorn, chips and salsa and candies.
- Do not eat anything after 7:00 pm. Don't forget to drink a glass of cold water before eating.
- Add lemon to your water. Lemon water can help you to lose weight because the sour taste helps your liver to get rid of toxins in your body. If your body is full of toxins, you will not lose weight period.

- This is a great one for all those people who don't like drinking water. Add some fruits to your cold ice water so that you can have a sweet flavor. Be careful of those flavors that say no added sugar because it can have high fructose corn syrup. You can add raspberry, strawberry, blueberry, oranges, pineapple, and grapes to name a few. Now, you have no excuse to not drink water. Drinking Kool-Aid is not the same thing as water because you added sugar. Try your fruit water you will love the delicious taste.

- You can make your salads in mason jars and carry with you on the go. Put the salad dressing to the bottom, and any veggie toppings you like. Then put your lettuce on the top. You will not have a soggy salad just pour the salad onto a plate and munch away.

- Try avoid keeping credit cards and cash on you. This will help to limit your spending on fast foods. When you have money in your possession, you will be more tempted to spend.

- Do a healthy vision board and hang it up where it can be visible to you daily. You can use photos out of healthy magazines or write on your board.

- Write on sticky notes and post them on your mirror, bedroom, fridge, garage, front, and back door. Doing this can help to remind you to drink water, take your lunch or snack with you and to exercise.

- Put the scale away after you weight yourself. Yes, the scale can be good and bad. When the scale doesn't move and you haven't lost any weight you get discourage and give up. Scales can vary so don't rely on them. Sometimes the best evidence of you losing weight is by your clothes. You can lose inches before you lose weight. Everyone body types are different and some people lose more weight than others do. While, some people lose more inches. You can measure your waist also with a measuring tape and keep track.

I hope these healthy tips can be of great assistance to you.

Good luck!

CHAPTER SEVEN

TASTY SMOOTHIES

As, you already know that smoothies are the bomb and incredibly delicious. Starting your day with a tasty glass of smoothie will do your body good. It will give you the energy that you need to jump-start your day because of all the nutrient value in your fruits and vegetables. Get in the habit of drinking smoothies daily will make your skin look flawless.

Here are some of my recipes that I would love to share with you. Only try these recipes after you have completed your detox. Hope you love these delicious smoothies.

Banana & Strawberry Twirl
½-cup strawberry

½ cup almond milk

Two bananas

½-teaspoon vanilla

Sprinkle of cinnamon

½-cup ice

Kale Berry Smash
½-cup kale

½-cup blueberry

½-cup raspberry

½-cup strawberry

1-cup ice

Passion
One kiwi

½-cup strawberry

½ cherry

½ raspberry

½-cup spinach

One apple

1-cup ice

Tropical Twist
One kiwi

½-cup pineapples

½-cup strawberry

½-cup blueberries

½ cup spinach

1 banana

1 cup ice

Mango Splash

1-cup mango

½-cup pineapples

½-cup peach

½-cup kale

1-cup ice

Sunshine

One grapefruit

½ pineapple

One orange

One peach

½-cup parsley

One lemon

1-cup ice

Veggie Blast

½-cup kale

½-cup spinach

One carrot

One celery stick

1-cup ice

Remember to blend your smoothie. If your smoothie is yucky looking then you need to add more ice your smoothie your body will love it.

CHAPTER EIGHT

HEALTHY JOURNEY

Now, that you've read this book it's time to begin your weight loss journey. I'm excited that you are taking this brave step. It will not be easy in the beginning, but it will be all worth it in the end.

Week One

Day One

- 2 cups spinach
- 1 cup kale
- 2 tbsp. flaxseed
- 1 cup blueberries
- 1 cup strawberries
- 1 apple
- 2 cups ice or water

Day Two

- 2 cups kale
- 1 cup peaches
- 1 cup mangoes
- 1 cup grapes
- 1 cup Swiss chard
- 2 tbsp. flaxseed
- 2 cups ice or water

Day Three

- 1 cup turnips
- 1 cup spinach
- 1 cup parsley
- 2 tbsp. flaxseed
- 1 cup pineapples
- 2 bananas
- 1 kiwi
- 2 cups ice or water

Day Four

- 1 cup spring mix
- 1 cup collard greens
- 1 cup kale
- 1 apple
- 2 tbsp. flaxseed
- 1 pear
- 1 cup peaches
- ½ cup grapes
- 2 cups ice or water

Day Five

- 2 cups spinach
- ¼ tsp cayenne pepper
- 1 cup parsley
- 2 celery sticks
- 1 cup blueberries
- 1 cup raspberries
- 1 apple
- 2 tbsp. flaxseed
- 2 cups ice or water

Day Six

- ½ cup collard greens
- 1 cup kale
- 1 cup spring mix
- ½ cup watercress
- 1 cup strawberries
- 1 ½ cup pineapples
- 1 cup mangoes
- 2 tbsp. flaxseed
- 2 cups ice or water

Day Seven

- 2 cups arugula
- 1 cup spinach
- 1 cup raspberries
- 1 pear
- 1 banana
- 1 apple
- 2 tbsp. flaxseed
- 2 cups ice or water

Day Eight

- ½ cup romaine lettuce
- 1 cup kale
- 1 cup Swiss chard
- ½ cup turnips
- 1 cup peaches
- 1 cup grapes
- 1 kiwi
- 2 tbsp. flaxseed
- 2 cups ice or water

Day Nine

- 2 cups parsley
- 1 cup mustard greens
- 1 cup pineapples
- 1 cup mangoes
- 2 apples
- 2 tbsp. flaxseed
- 2 cups ice or water

Day Ten

- 2 cups spring mix
- 1 cup spinach
- 1 cup blueberries
- 1 cup strawberries
- ½ raspberries
- 2 tbsp. flaxseeds
- 2 cups ice or water

You will only be doing a green smoothie for 10 days. Try to push to ten days; you can do it. You can add 1 scoop of protein powder to your smoothies. Try organic protein. If you have frozen fruits you can use water, but if you're using fresh fruits use ice to blend. Using large blenders will hold all of the ingredients. If you have a smaller blender, divide your ingredients. Preparing your smoothies the night before or a few days in advance can save you lots of time. Separate your vegetables and fruits in bags or containers. You can freeze your smoothie bags for the week, take out the night before, and refrigerate the bag. Smoothies can be put into fridge for a later time. Do not use any smoothies for the following day.

Here are some helpful tips:

- Get adequate sleep.
- Use this time to relax. Don't over work yourself.
- No alcohol or any solid foods.
- Drink eight glasses of water with ½ teaspoon of ginger, 10 mint leaves, 10 cucumber slices, and 1 lemon. Steep water overnight to get a great diffuse.
- Only one fruit per day for a snack. (½ cup of blueberries, 6 strawberries, 1 apple, 1 grapefruit, ½ cup raspberries) Rotate your fruits daily.
- Only two snacks per day.
- Unsweetened peanut butter 2 tbsp., ¼-cup almonds unsalted, 10 slices cucumbers, six celery sticks, six carrot sticks, unsalted pecans 1 handful. Choose only one per day.

- You can drink 12-16 ounces of smoothies 3 times a day breakfast, lunch, dinner. If you feel too full, drink your smoothies for snack. Make sure blend your smoothies well.
- If you get any headaches, drink more water or eat an apple and rest.
- No exercise during cleanse as you will be on a c
- During your cleansed is a great time to meditate.
- Find something to occupy your time so you don't think about food.
- Flaxseed will help to keep you full longer.
- Stay away from sugar. The only sugar should come from your fruits.

Week Two Next Five Days

This week you will start gradually eating again, but a lot healthier.

- Green smoothie of choice for breakfast with less ingredients. (¼ cup parsley, ¼-cup kale, ¼-

cup blueberries, ½-cup spinach, ½-cup raspberries, ½ tbsp. flaxseed, ½-cup water, or ice).

- You can eat one grapefruit.
- Drink diffused water as mentioned earlier 8 cups.
- Lunch small romaine salad with homemade dressing, one can tuna, squeeze lemon, or kale salad w/cherry tomatoes, celery, cucumbers, and boiled eggs. No cheese.
- No sugar or junk food
- Two glasses grapefruit juice. No store juice. Make your own juice fresh.
- Snacks are the same as week one. One of each. No more than two snacks per day.
- For dinner you can have fish, salmon, shrimp, chicken breast, tofu, lean red meat, turkey. Only choose one 4oz a day with two choices of vegetables (spinach, collard greens, swiss chard, arugula, kale, peas, broccoli, black beans, green beans etc). No added seasoning with sodium. Use natural herbs and Mrs. Dash. No fried food,

sauces, or butter. Eat bake, sautéed, grilled, or boiled. Do not eat red meat more than once a week.

- Drink a glass of water before meals and snacks. This helps to make you fuller.

Keep going you're almost done. PUSH!

Week Three Last Five Days

Breakfast choices choose only one option.
- Green smoothie for breakfast or lunch.
- One cup oatmeal no added sugar 1 tsp natural honey, cinnamon or sprinkle of almonds, 6 dices of apples on top. One fruit orange, ½-cup grapes, blueberries, or your choice. This is breakfast.
- Two boil eggs and a fruit of choice for breakfast.
- One low fat yogurt and a boil egg for breakfast.
- Egg omelet with spinach no butter, olive oil only.

- Drink a glass of grapefruit juice daily.

For lunch and dinner, choose one option from week two. Do not eat the same meat 2 times a day. Eat only 4oz of protein for lunch and dinner. Two choices of vegetables with no oil. Red meat no more than two times per week as it takes longer to digest. If you still feel hungry, drink a glass of water.

- 2-3 snacks a day fruit and a healthy snack any choice listed in week 2. Do not eat the same snack in one day. The third snack can be eaten as a dessert a handful of blueberries or an apple.
- No desserts such as cakes, cookies.
- You can add exercise to your regimen 2-4 times a week. This will help you to maintain your weight, stay fit, fabulous and in shape.

Remember to stay on track. You survived and I am so proud of you. As you start adding carbs back to your diet, the key is to choose healthy ones and eat in moderation. Overeating can cause you to gain weight right back and you don't want this to happen. Eating more calories than allowed can cause you to put on pounds. Look in the mirror and say this weight is off forever. Don't eat pasta or rice every day. When you eat out do it on occasions and make healthy choices. You have come too far to go back to your old unhealthy eating habits. This is a long-term journey lifestyle change. Now, you can go out with the girls and go shopping for that new outfit you've been waiting for a long time to wear. Send me a picture and your success story to my Healthy N Fabulous group page on facebook. You are now healthy and fabulous and living a healthy lifestyle.

Congratulations!

Heathy N Fabulous Quiz

Answering these questions can help you to see where you're making mistakes.

1.   Why do you want to lose weight?

_____

_____

_____

_____

2.   How much weight are you trying to lose?

_____

3.   What is your ideal weight goal?

_____

4.   What foods do you crave the most and why?

_____

_____

_____

_____

5.   What steps can you take to help you eliminate your cravings?

_____

_____

_____

_____

6.   Do you snack late at night?

_____

7.   Do you exercise?

_____

8.   How many times per week do you exercise?

_____

9.   How many times per week do you eat out?

_____

10.   Is food your comfort when you're sad?

_____

11.   List three things that you can do to help you cope instead of overeating.

_____, _____,

_____.

12.   Do you eat fruits and vegetables?

_____

13.   How many times per week do you eat fruits and vegetables?

_____

14.   How many glasses of water do you drink per day?

_____

15.   How many hours of sleep do you get at night?

_____

16.   Are you willing to make a healthy lifestyle change?

_____

17.   Do you have any health issues?

_____

18.   Will you quit when you get tired?

_____

Now that you've answered these questions, you can make the necessary changes that you need to.

CHAPTER NINE

HEALTHY N FABULOUS AFFIRMATIONS

✓   I love me.

✓   I am super woman.

✓   I can achieve my weight goal.

✓   I am proud of my progress.

✓   I have the power and strength to finish strong.

✓   Exercise is a part of my life now.

✓   From this day forward, I will live a healthy lifestyle.

✓   I will not eat unhealthy foods.

✓   I will eat healthy forever.

✓   I will only eat unhealthy on special occasions and in moderation.

✓   I will take care of my health.

✓   I love my body.

✓   I am beautiful.

✓   I am Healthy N Fabulous.

CHAPTER TEN

HEALTHY GROCERY LIST

FRUITS
APPLE

ORANGE

MANGO

PINEAPPLE

PEACH

GRAPE

BANANA

BLUEBERRY

RASPBERRY

WATERMELON

KIWI

COCONUT

CHERRY

PEAR

CANTALOUPE

STRAWBERRY

VEGETABLES
SPINACH

BROCCOLI

KALE

TURNIPS

TOMATOES

GREEN PEPPERS

ONIONS

GARLIC

GREEN BEANS

COLLARD- GREENS

ROMAINE- LETTUCE

SPRING MIX LETTUCE

CHICKPEAS

KIDNEY BEANS

BLACK BEANS

PARSLEY

ASPARAGUS

PEAS

BASIL LEAF

CABBAGE

OKRA

AVOCADO

WATERCRESS

MUSTARD-GREENS

ARUGULA

SWISS CHARD

SQUASH

ZUCCHINI

CARBS

COTTAGE CHEESE

QUINOA

WHEAT BREAD/PASTA

MISC. ITEMS

HEMP SEEDS

OLIVE OIL

GRAPESEED- OIL

COCONUT OIL

MRS. DASH

THYME

RED PEPPER

OLIVES

CAYENNE -PEPPER

CINNAMON

NATURAL- RAW HONEY

STEVIA

APPLE CIDER-VINEGAR

NATURAL-HER

PROTEINS

FISH

EGGS

TOFU

TURKEY

SKIM MILK

ALMOND MILK

OATS

EGG PLANT

CHICKEN BREAST

TUNA

WHEY PROTEIN

HEMP PROTEIN

RICE PROTEIN

SNACKS

UNSWEETENED PEANUT- BUTTER

ALMOND

UNSALTED- NUTS

CUCUMBER

CELERY

CARROT

BROCCOLI

LOW FAT- YOGURT

SUNFLOWER-SEED

PISTACHIO-SEED

CHIA-SEED

FLAXSEED

CHERRY- TOMATOES

PECANS

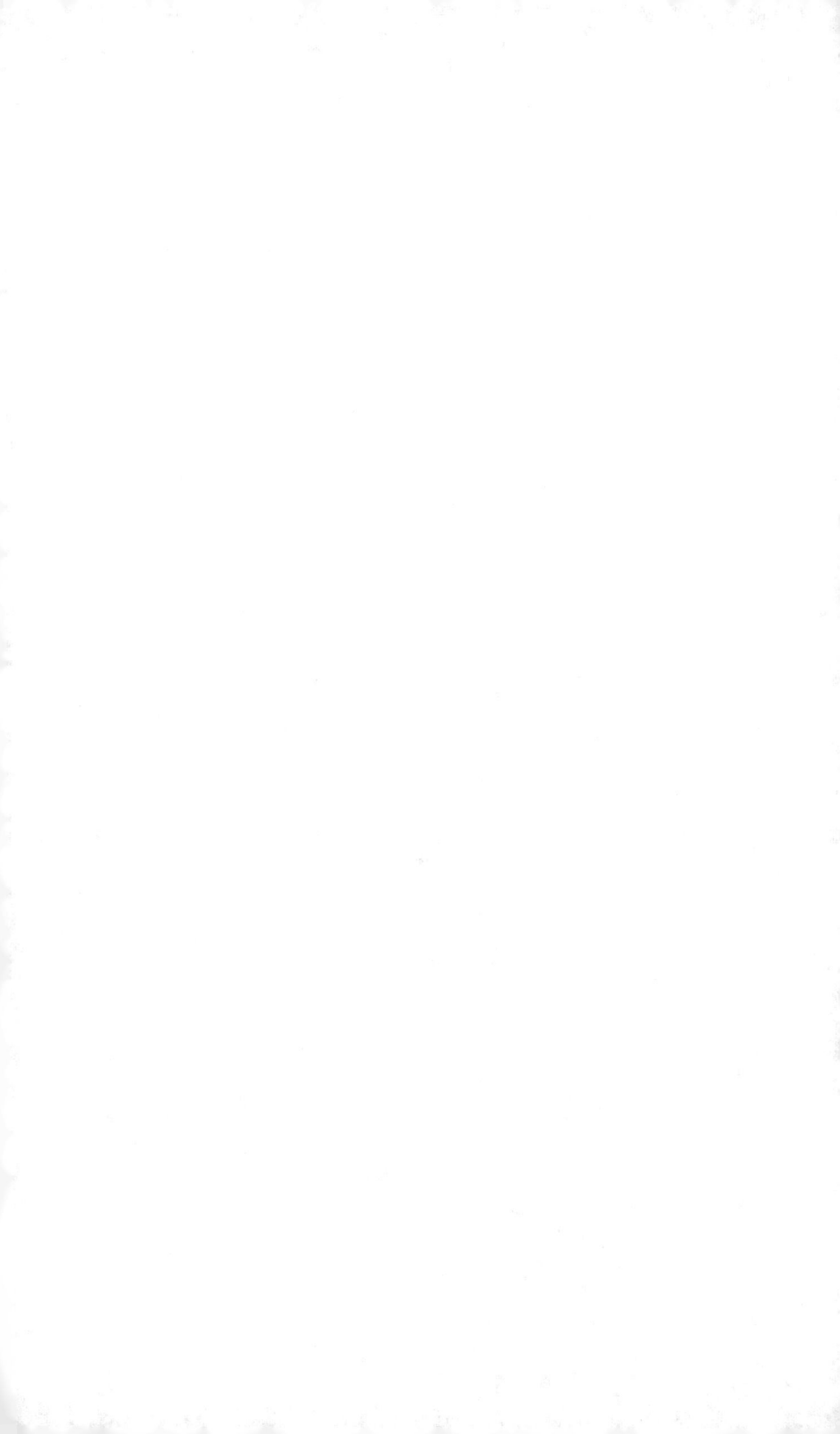

www.ingramcontent.com/pod-product-compliance
Lightning Source LLC
Chambersburg PA
CBHW071212280526
45787CB00002B/652